Alkaline Ketogenic Mix
Quick, Easy and Delicious Recipes & Tips for Natural Weight Loss and a Healthy Lifestyle

By Elena Garcia

Copyright Elena Garcia © 2019

Sign up for new books, fresh tips, super healthy recipes, and our latest wellness releases:

www.YourWellnessBooks.com

Disclaimer

A physician has not written the information in this book. It is advisable that you visit a qualified dietician so that you can obtain a highly personalized treatment for your case, especially if you want to lose weight effectively. This book is for informational and educational purposes only and is not intended for medical purposes. Please consult your physician before making any drastic changes to your diet.

All information in this book has been carefully researched and checked for factual accuracy. However, the author and publishers make no warranty, expressed or implied, that the information contained herein is appropriate for every individual, situation or purpose, and assume no responsibility for errors or omission. The reader assumes the risk, and full responsibility for all actions and the author will not be held liable for any loss or damage, whether consequential, incidental, and special or otherwise, that may result from the information presented in this publication.

2

The book is not intended to provide medical advice or to take the place of medical advice and treatment from your personal physician. Readers are advised to consult their own doctors or other qualified health professionals regarding the treatment of medical conditions. The author shall not be held liable or responsible for any misunderstanding or misuse of the information contained in this book. The information is not intended to diagnose, treat, or cure any disease.

If you suffer from any medical condition, are pregnant, lactating, or on medication, be sure to talk to your doctor before making any drastic changes in your diet and lifestyle.

Contents

Introduction

Thank You for purchasing this book.
It means you are very serious about your health and wellbeing.

Whether your goal is to lose weight, enjoy more energy, or learn a few delicious healing recipes- you have come to the right place.

You are probably thinking...what? Alkaline- Ketogenic Mix? What kind of diet is that? Can I do it? Is it easy to follow? What do the recipes look like? Are they tasty?

Don't worry. Even if you are a total beginner, and never heard of the keto or alkaline diets, this book will guide you in the right direction.

It's because it is designed for busy people, like you and many others. People who are looking for something simple and effective to follow.

I originally created this guide for my family and friends, because everyone was curious about my own transformation and what I was eating. After realizing how much success my family and friends had with this "hybrid" diet, I knew I could not keep this guide to myself. I wanted to turn it into an easily accessible and affordable program you can jump in and experience all the fantastic health and wellness benefits yourself. And so, I decided to write this little booklet.

Here is precisely what you can expect:

- First, I will introduce you to all the benefits of the alkaline – ketogenic hybrid diet. That will help you get and stay motivated to take massive-inspired action.
- Then, we will dive into an elementary science and practice behind both diets, so that you understand the basics and know what to do without feeling overwhelmed.
- We will also go through certain precautions and common beginner mistakes to avoid. I don't want you to waste your time.

Proper preparation is critical.

-To be successful with this diet, you need to know what to eat, what to avoid, and what you can enjoy in moderation. In this part, you will get very detailed food lists. You will be very positively surprised how many delicious foods you can enjoy on this diet.
And don't worry! You will not feel hungry or deprived (not at all).

-Finally, you will get a ton of super healthy recipes that fuse the best of alkaline and ketogenic diets. You will get quick and delicious recipes for breakfast, lunch, and dinner as well as snacks. This book is not like a strict program, it's more of a flexible guide, where you can choose your favorite recipes and combine them the way you want. The reason being- if there is a recipe you don't like, and you would need to stick to it, you would lose your motivation. The approach I want to take is freedom and flexibility, while still enjoying, your strong alkaline ketogenic foundation.

So, feel free to pick and choose and enjoy your favorite breakfast, lunch, and dinner recipes! Some recipes can also be used as a template to create your own. It may take some time, so at first, you will find the tips helpful. After you have gotten the hang of it, you will know the right food combinations. Then, you will be able to come up with your own recipes, even with your eyes closed.

Ready to transform? Let's do this. I am so excited you are here! Whatever stage you're at, you are in the right place. If you are just starting out, this guide will be a great "shortcut."

If you are not new to this way of eating, it will inspire you even more and help you optimize your efforts.

After experiencing results and transformation yourself, share this guide with your family and friends to help them too. Everyone deserves to know this information.

Let's start off with keto...what exactly is it? Is the ketogenic diet some new fad?

While the keto diet is definitely more popular these days, it's not a fad. In fact, it's been around for thousands of years, and this is how our ancestors would eat- combining animal products and good fats with some vegetables and herbs.

This is precisely what we will be doing through this guide! We will be embracing the best of the alkaline diet (a ton of fresh nutrient-packed veggies and other healing plant-based foods) with the best of the ketogenic diet (good fats, healthy animal products, and lean protein).

The ketogenic diet has been used clinically since early 1900, to help people with epilepsy.

So what exactly is it?

The simplest definition is:

The ketogenic diet is a diet low in carbs and high in healthy fats.

It encourages to massively reduce the carbohydrate intake and replace it with good, healthy fats (more on healthy vs. unhealthy fats later). This cutback in carbs puts your body into a metabolic state called ketosis.

When in ketosis, your body becomes super-efficient at burning fat for energy. A ketogenic diet can also help reduce blood sugar and insulin levels.

The fact is that we are designed to have periods where we "fast from carbs" and when our glucose levels are depleted.

Then, we start using our body very cleverly, using ketones for fuel. Ketones are the result of our body burning fat for food. The liver converts body fats and ingested fats into ketones.

Transition your diet into a more keto-friendly diet, it's straightforward. It means fewer sugars and carbs and more good fats while eating well!

Following this simple rule (even without going keto full-time) will help you transform your health. It will also help you lose weight naturally if you stay committed to it.

You will no longer be hooked on all those "crappy carbs" and with the new "keto energy" you will feel much more motivated to work out and be more active.

The problem is that in this day and age we eat way too many carbs and sugars. To make it even worse, we eat processed carbs and sugars (pasta, candy, cakes, etc.). Most people find it hard to start their day without carbs and sugar.

Luckily, once you get into the ketogenic lifestyle, your body is using fat for fuel. The first few days may be a bit weird, but it's like anything, if you give up smoking, drinking...you will feel weird because you are getting rid of toxins. But, looking at the long-term benefits, a ketogenic friendly lifestyle really makes sense as it:

-manages your sugar levels, prevents diabetes

-normalizes your hormones and auto-immune system

-is great for neurological health

-has even been used in clinical settings to prevent Alzheimer's, epilepsies, type 3 diabetes

Also, your brain will thrive. While it can use both glucose and fats for fuel, ketones are a really clean energy source. I can now concentrate much better and for much longer, while feeling less tired because I have transitioned my diet in a more ketogenic friendly direction.

I can now enjoy much more mental clarity; there is no brain fog.

Here are other benefits of aligning your dietary choices with a ketogenic-friendly way:

-you will experience reduced hunger and reduced cravings

-you will be burning fat and reducing carbs and so normalizing your insulin levels

-you will protect your heart while raising the good cholesterol

-you will enjoy the anti-age benefits, as keto foods promote longevity and vitality (while nobody ever promised us we will live forever, by making a decision to stay healthy, we make sure that the time we are here on earth, we feel good and are vibrant).

In other words- burning crappy carbs for energy is like burning dirty fuel while burning fat is a much cleaner fuel while avoiding brain fog. In fact, your brain thrives on ketones.

So here's what the ketogenic diet consists of:

-75%- 80% fat (don't worry, it's all good fat and will not make you fat).

-5-15% healthy, clean protein

-5% good, unprocessed carbs (yea, you can still eat some carbs and the carbs we will be focusing on, will be healthy unprocessed no sugar carbs so no worries, there is no starvation involved here).

While it may seem like something hard to follow, especially when you still got that pasta meal on your mind, it will all become effortless after you get into the creamy, fatty, and actually guilt-free ketogenic friendly recipes!

My personal story

After focusing on ketogenic friendly foods and a diet rich in greens and alkaline vegetables, I now have more time in my day. Yes! It's because I am less focused on food, I can use that energy to focus on my family, and activities I am passionate about. I even felt inspired to join yoga classes (and I feel motivated to attend them regularly).

I no longer crave sugar. Yes, every now and then I add some fruit to my diet (like a smoothie or a home-made fruity ice cream). When there is a family occasion, I have a "little dessert". As an exception.

Usually, I eat the keto-friendly way during the week, and as I said before, since I no longer crave sugar all the time and I feel more energized, it feels like I have more free time. I am also less moody, and I no longer experience menstrual cramps and headaches (so I gain a few "extra days" of life each and every month).

On the weekends, I still enjoy my alkaline keto diet, but sometimes I allow myself to have some rice when we go out for Thai food, or some other foods that are off the alkaline keto list. Hey, a little treat every now and then is OK!

It's a great emotional relief to know, I am in the drivers' seat, I choose some "cheat" foods every now, and then I don't have to give them all up forever. But, I know I have my "healthy foundation," and I am moving forward with my goals.

At the same time, I already have a list of local restaurants where I know I can order meals that are both alkaline and keto friendly, and in this book, I will share my best tips and tricks with you too. It's really not that hard to follow, and once you have started experiencing all the benefits, you will want to tell everyone about it.

It may not even be necessary as your results will speak for themselves, and everyone will be curious to know your diet.

You can do it too it's up to you if you want to be strictly alkaline-keto or simply eat this way most of the time, which is way easier for most people.

The good news is that it's not about perfection, so never beat yourself up for not following through 100%.

Treat it as a learning experience to get in touch with your body, observe your energy and mood, and learn some super delicious and healthy recipes. This book can also be used as a "part-time" guide.

Also, it's not about putting labels and names on you and what you eat. The labels are simply designed as some guidelines so that we feel inspired to create our foundation of vibrant health.

This is what this book is all about. I want to share with you the best of the alkaline and keto diets. I want you to feel inspired to create a healthy lifestyle you enjoy, a lifestyle that is sustainable so that it doesn't feel like another diet to "stick to."

So now that we have covered the basics of the keto diet let's have a look at the alkaline diet.

***

If you have read my other books: *Alkaline Paleo Mix,* and/or *Alkaline Diet,* you may choose to skip this part of the book and dive straight into Alkaline Keto food lists.

•••

What is the alkaline diet?

"Going green" is the way to describe an alkaline diet and lifestyle because the focus is on green vegetables in general, as they are the most alkaline food you can ingest.

The benefits of the alkaline diet are numerous. Let us name a few:

WEIGHT LOSS

An alkaline diet will assist you in losing weight. One way that it does this is obvious. The foods you will be eating are very healthy, rich in minerals and low calorie in general.

You will also be reducing the amount of acid in your body. The body stores fat to protect itself from an abundance of acid. It is a self-preservation method. This is part of the reason why people who exercise a lot and drink an excess of caffeine cannot seem to lose those extra pounds. Their bodies are clinging to that fat to minimize the effects of all of the acid in their systems. Caffeine is really acid-forming, and it's not the most sustainable source of energy. That is why we recommend you drink it in moderation, for your own enjoyment rather than a source of energy you depend on.

Another benefit of an alkaline lifestyle regarding weight loss is that alkaline systems have more oxygen in their cells. Oxygen is a very essential part of eliminating fat cells from the body. The more oxygen in your system, the more efficient your metabolism will be.

ENERGY

Before my "healthy alkaline transformation," caffeine was my buddy. I am half-Spanish and half-Italian, and so drinking coffee is deeply rooted in my culture.

I started drinking coffee when I was only eleven. Everyone drinks coffee in Italy, where I grew up. People socialize drinking coffee in the streets. Everyone is always up for a cappuccino or espresso. Most of the Italians would even tell you that coffee is super healthy. While I do agree that having a nice cup of coffee is great as a treat, we should not depend on it for energy. Moderation is the key.

Well, thanks to my new alkaline lifestyle, I have totally changed my attitude and managed to control my caffeine addiction. I was one of those people who did not even want to converse until I had downed my first cup of coffee. I thought that I was simply hormonal or sleep deprived. I always envied other people who had a constant supply of energy. Little did I know that an alkaline lifestyle could provide that for me!

Going green does not only give you energy for the apparent reason that you are eating many more healthy, energizing vitamins. You are negating the acid-induced lethargy that is brought on by an unhealthy acid-forming diet.

Not only do our bodies need an abundance of oxygen to lose weight, but we also need oxygen in our cells to energize us. The lack of oxygen in our cells causes fatigue. No, it is not just because you worked too late or partied to hard the night before. It is internal. If your cells are trying to function in a highly acidic environment, they will not be able to transfer oxygen efficiently; leading of course to exhaustion.

Cells in the body also make something that is called adenosine triphosphate (ATP). If your system is very acidic, it harms the ability of your cells to produce it. In the scientific world, it is known as the "energy currency of life." The ATP molecule contains the energy that we need to accomplish most things that we do (both internally and externally).

BODILY FUNCTIONS

Another benefit of the alkaline lifestyle is that your body will be able to function at an optimum level instead of being inhibited by acids:

- Your heartbeat is thrown off by acidic wastes in the body. The stomach suffers greatly from over-acidity.

- The liver's job is to get rid of acid toxins, but also to produce alkaline enzymes. By simply reducing your acid intake, you can internally boost your alkalinity thanks to your liver!

- Your pancreas thrives on alkalinity. Too much acid in your system throws off your pancreas. If you eat alkaline foods, your pancreas can regulate your blood sugars.

- Your kidneys also help to keep your body alkaline. When they are overwhelmed by an acidic diet, they cannot do their job

- The lymph fluids function most efficiently in an alkaline system. They remove acid waste. Acidic systems not only have a slower lymph flow causing acids to be stored; they can also cause acids to be reabsorbed through lymphatic ducts in your intestines that would typically be excreted.

MENTAL FOCUS

The alkalinity of the system is one of the best ways to focus and strengthen the mind. Just as the rest of the body is poorly affected by acid-forming foods and other toxins, so is your brain. And as we all know, it should be possible to control your emotions and decision making with your mind. Guess what? If your body is too acidic and is not alkaline, your mental clarity will be cloudy, your decision making could be off, as well as your emotional state.

DETOX

Another huge benefit of an alkaline lifestyle is detoxification. First, you are going to be cutting out processed foods that are continually adding toxins to your system.

Secondly, you are going to be eating foods that allow your body to detox and rid itself of the acids that have built up in your system all this time. When we detoxify our bodies, our emotions, bodily functions, and mental functions are able to operate at their optimum levels.

The number of benefits that come with living alkaline are numerous. As you help your body rebalance its optimal blood pH, you will find, as we did, that you have never felt better. We are still seeing improvement and reaping the rewards of this holistic approach to not only eating alkaline foods but living alkaline.

Alkaline vs. Acidic? Sounds like the title fight for a lightweight boxing match. In reality, it is a fight, a fight for the pH balance of your body. pH levels are basically the measure of how acidic a liquid is.

Our bodies function optimally when our blood is at about 7.35 -7.45 pH.

pH levels range from 0 to 14. 0 is the highest level of acidity, but basically, everything 0-7 would be considered acidic. The 7-14 range is alkaline.

Before we dive into complicated pH discussions, here is one thing to understand:

-The alkaline <u>diet is not about changing or "raising" your pH</u>. This is where many alkaline guides go wrong. You see, our body is smart enough to **self-regulate** our pH for us, no matter what we eat.

Unfortunately, when you constantly bombard your body with acid-forming foods (for example processed foods, fast food, alcohol, sugar, and even too much meat) you torture your body with incredible stress. Why? Well because it has to work harder to maintain that optimal pH...

Here's simple example...

Imagine you immerse yourself in a bath filled with ice. You say, but hey, my body can self-regulate its optimal temperature, right? And yes, it can. But it will eventually collapse, and you will get ill. The same happens with nutrition and our blood pH.

You can spend years indulging in toxic, processed, acid-forming foods that only deprive your body of its vital nutrients, saying: "But hey, my body will self-regulate its optimal blood pH."

And again, it will...but sooner or later it will give up and manifest a disease. It will accumulate fat as its natural defense function to protect your body from over-acidity. We don't wanna end up there, right?

So, to sum up- the alkaline diet is a natural, holistic system, a nutritional lifestyle that advocates the consumption of fresh, unprocessed foods that are rich in nutrients. These are called alkaline foods, and they help your body stimulate its optimal healing functions. Yes! A healthy body needs nutrients, and fresh fruits and vegetables are great for that.

The problem is that nowadays, most diets are filled with acid-forming foods that eventually make it hard for the body to regulate its optimal, healthy blood pH. Acidosis is very common in this day and age thanks to things we drink as well: coffee, alcohol, sugar, crappy carbs, and sodas all have an acidic effect on our bodies. Not to mention the chemicals many people take in through things like smoking and drugs (even prescription drugs have this effect).

There are many ways that you could become acidic. Eating acid-forming foods, stress, taking in too many toxins, and bodily processes all cause acidity in the body. Our internal systems try to balance themselves out and bring pH up with the help of alkaline minerals that we can ingest through our diet. If we do not take in a higher percentage of alkaline than acidic foods, we can become too acidic.

When you are acidic, it makes every process that your body does typically much more difficult or impossible for it to accomplish. We cannot absorb the beneficial nutrients we need from our food correctly. Our cells are not able to produce energy efficiently.

Our bodies are not able to fix damaged cells properly. We will not be able to detoxify properly. Fatigue and illness will drag you down. Sounds horrible; does it not? Here are some signs that you are overly acidic:

- ✓ Feeling tired all the time. You have no physical or mental drive at all.

- ✓ You always feel cold.

- ✓ You get sick easily.

✓ You are depressed or just feel "blah" all the time for no real reason

✓ You are easily overstimulated and stressed by noise, light, etc.

✓ You get headaches for no apparent reason

✓ You get watery eyes or inflamed eyelids.

✓ Your teeth are sensitive and may crack or chip

✓ Your gums are inflamed, and you are susceptible to canker sores

✓ You have recurring bouts with throat problems including tonsillitis

✓ Acidic stomach with acid indigestion and reflux is always an issue

✓ Your fingernails crack, split, and break

✓ You have super dry hair that sheds and is hay-like with split ends

✓ You have dry, ashy skin

✓ Your skin breaks out in acne or is irritated when you sweat

✓ You get leg cramps and spasms (this includes restless leg syndrome).

(Of course, remember that whenever you experience any health/medical conditions, you need to see your doctor first and get a checkup.)

Changing your diet to one that is full of alkaline foods is one of the easiest and best things you can do for your overall health. I was so ecstatic that I did! And the best thing is- we will be combining alkaline foods with keto friendly meals to make it easy, delicious and fun! Much simpler to follow for the long term.

But the way we see it is this- it's perfect! Plus, it's not a diet, it's a lifestyle.

What I really like about the alkaline diet is that you don't have to be 100% perfect. It's enough to make sure you add a ton of greens and veggies and make your diet rich in alkaline foods.

It's easy to do when you focus on serving your lunch or dinner with a big green salad or start drinking green juices (I will show you how to go about it in the recipe section later).

When it comes to the alkaline diet, there is something called the 70/30 rule meaning that about 70% of your diet should be fresh, nutrient dense alkaline-forming foods and the remaining 30% can be acid- forming foods (however they still should be clean and organic, for example, grass-fed meat or organic eggs).

This is what we will be doing in this book. For example, for breakfast, you can enjoy scrambled eggs, made with coconut oil or fresh butter, with some organic goat cheese and spices. You can serve it on a big heap of fresh spinach or arugula leaves with some green juice.

That will give you a ton of energy- green foods and veggies will help you add fresh nutrients into your diet while eggs and some lean protein and good fats will keep you full. You will no longer crave crappy carbs or sugars.

Or...imagine, some fresh salmon, served with a large avocado, lime juice, and spices.

Or...an amazing veggie salad with some naughty bacon and organic cheese.

The basic rule to shift your meals towards an alkaline-keto friendly style is to:

-add more greens to your diet (can be done through salads, or you can juice the greens, or add them to your smoothies).

-add more good fats (for example: organic cheese, fish, avocado, coconut oil)

Now, let's have a break from the theory and have a look at the keto food lists. Then, we will have a closer look at the alkaline foods and their role in this lifestyle. The goal is to help you have more energy, enjoy better vitality, and feel fabulous.

Your alkaline-keto-friendly food lists

The following foods can be eaten to your heart's content!

Oh, and when it comes to eating meat, you can choose fattier cuts with skin and on the bone. In fact, you totally should!

When choosing fish, choose all wild-caught fish with fins and scales. Industrial fish is full of toxins and not good for you.

All kinds of veggies are excellent and making sure you serve your keto meals on heaps of greens will help you stay fully nourished and prevent sugar cravings too.

Also, please note that the food lists below are designed for an average, busy person who simply wishes to stay healthy, energized, or lose some weight. So, they are a bit simplified. If you have any specific goals, whether it's athletic, or healing any particular health issue, I would recommend you invest in a dietician specializing in ketogenic diets and alkaline foods so that they can create personalized food lists for you and your desired outcome.

Keto - Meat (try to go for organic)

• Beef

• Lamb

• Turkey

• Duck

• Chicken

• Goat

• Venison

• Veal

• Buffalo

• Elk

• As well as **all organ meats such as liver, kidney, etc.** of above animals

Keto - Fish (try to go for freshly caught)

- Salmon
- Mackerel
- tuna
- haddock
- halibut
- bass
- trout
- sole
- herring
- snapper
- sardines
- whitefish
- whiting

+ as well as a roe from any of these fish

+All kinds of bone broths and stocks of above meat and fish are allowed

+ Dried and cured meats from the above-mentioned animals and fish are allowed

Keto - Eggs and Dairy Products

- organic free-range chicken eggs
- duck and goose organic free-range eggs
- raw full-fat cheeses
- raw cream
- all types of kefir - Raw or organic
- pasteurized cow's milk, goat's milk
- sheep's milk

- *Please note- Dairy products can be skipped if you are lactose intolerant. Most recipes from this book use plant-based milk that is both alkaline and keto friendly (coconut milk, almond milk, etc.)*

It's really up to you. Personally, I like to have a little bit of organic cheese or organic kefir every now and then. But, most of the time, I live a dairy-free lifestyle.

Alkaline Keto Veggies

- **All green leafy vegetables:**
- Spinach
- Kale
- swiss chard
- chicory
- romaine and iceberg lettuce
- little gem
- radicchio
- dandelion
- lettuce
- greens,
- chives
- lettuce
- bok choy
- mustard greens
- turnip greens
- nasturtium
- watercress,
- rocket/arugula

- Micro-greens seed sprouts
- Bell pepper

All cruciferous vegetables:

- broccoli
- cabbage
- radish
- kohlrabi
- horseradish
- daikon
- collard greens
- cauliflower
- brussels sprouts
- spring greens

Other non-starchy vegetables:

- artichoke
- asparagus
- avocado
- celery
- endive
- fennel
- garlic
- garlic

Herbs

- Basil
- Cilantro

- Mint
- parsley

Other:

- kelp
- leeks
- okra
- olives
- onion
- spring/green onions
- water
- shallots
- mushrooms (not considered alkaline by most alkaline experts, however, can be added in small amounts and are still keto friendly).
- chestnuts

Alkaline Grasses

- wheatgrass juice
- barley grass juice

Healthy Keto Fats & Oils (the ones coming from plants are also alkaline)

• Extra-virgin coconut oil

• Extra virgin olive oil (not for cooking)

• Raw butter or ghee

- Grass-fed pasteurized butter or ghee

- Beef tallow

- Goat's milk butter (not for cooking)

- Coconut milk cream (organic, with no additives)

- Coconut butter

Condiments

- All kinds of organic spices, herbs, and pepper

- Unrefined sea salt, Himalaya salt, and rock salt

- Organic Mustard (with no artificial additives)

- Organic Apple cider vinegar

- Balsamic vinegar (with no artificial additives)

- Organic Mayonnaise (made with only natural

oils, no vegetable oil)

- Fresh home-made guacamole

Keto Friendly Fermented Foods

- Raw, lacto-fermented sauerkraut

- Raw, lacto-fermented kimchi

- Dairy probiotic foods listed - such as kefir and raw milk products

- Pickled vegetables (must be raw, lactofermented)

Drinks

- Filtered water
- Alkaline water
- Herbal infusions (caffeine-free)
- Sparkling mineral water
- Bone broth
- Filtered water with fresh lemon or lime
- Green juice with no high sugar fruit in it (for example celery juice, kale juice, wheat grass juice)

Low Sugar Alkaline & Keto Fruit:

- limes
- lemons
- grapefruits
- pomegranates
- blueberries

Fats & Oils

• Flax oil (not for cooking)

• Avocado oil (not for cooking)

• Hemp seed oil (not for cooking)

• Walnut oil (not for cooking)

• Expeller-pressed sesame oil (not for cooking)

• Duck fat

- Goose fat

Nuts & Seeds

- Flaxseed (raw, ground)

- Sesame seeds

- Tahini (sesame butter)

- Almonds (raw, soaked/sprouted)

- Almond butter

- Brazils (raw, soaked/sprouted)

- Hazelnuts (raw, soaked/sprouted)

- Pecans (raw, soaked/sprouted)

- Pistachio Nuts (raw, soaked/sprouted)

- Walnuts (raw, soaked/sprouted)

- Macadamias (raw, soaked/sprouted)

- Macadamia butter

- Pine Nuts

- Pili nuts

- Chia seeds (raw and soaked)

- Nut flours - Coconut, almond

I think it's pretty good news so far?

Have you noticed how the "eat freely" food lists combine organic animal products, good fats and super healthy, chlorophyll-rich alkaline-forming veggies?

Their goal is to help your body get back in balance naturally.

We will talk in detail about those veggies later. I will also share with you some tips and recipes to make sure you eat enough of them. So even if you are not a veggie person, don't worry. We got you covered.

To sum up the first series of our food lists, the foods that are freely allowed, I cannot help myself but to make this remark...

My Mediterranean grandma, who lived (enjoying very good health) till 95 years old, used a lot of healthy food combinations from the lists above, for example:

-fresh salmon with a ton of green veggies, drizzled with organic olive oil (I can still remember how everyone would criticize her for "adding more fat," but she was adding good fat)

-hard boiled eggs with fresh lettuce, tomato, avocado and olive oil, herbs and sea salt

-organic meat with a ton of leafy greens

-bone broths with good fats in it

-scrambled eggs, with herbs, butter, and leafy greens

-fresh tuna salad with olive oil and apple cider vinegar

-avocado salad with olive oil, herbs, sea salt, and lemon juice

-full-fat cheese with veggies, olives, and good oils, as a salad...

I am getting hungry now when I look at that menu!

My grandma was also a fan of lemon-infused water as well as adding a bit of apple cider vinegar to water and having it as a night drink. I do it all the time, it's a healthy habit to develop, and it helps reduce inflammation (inflammation is the root of all evil).

Ok, so now after we have seen what is allowed on this lifestyle and how delicious it can get, let's focus on the second part of the food lists. Please note, it will not be hard to eliminate or reduce them, after you have started adding the "freely allowed" foods. Give your body what it needs to thrive, and there will be less and less unwanted food cravings.

Foods to AVOID as much as possible:

Sugars, Sweeteners & Other

- White and brown sugar
- Coconut sugar
- Chocolate
- Raw honey
- Date syrup
- Pure maple syrup
- Molasses
- Tropical fruits
- Fruit juice
- Candy

Drinks

- Alcohol

- Caffeine
- A note about caffeine: 1 quality expresso a day is fine if you really need it. If you do, be sure to stay hydrated throughout the day. My delicious alkaline keto drinks from the recipe section will help you with that.

Other foods and drinks to avoid:

All commercial, refined, heat-treated,

denatured or artificial foods such as:

- breads
- baked goods
- sauces
- pastries,
- tinned foods
- microwave meals
- fast food
- breakfast cereals
- confectionery,
- sweets
- soy
- processed milk

Other:

All artificial sweeteners:

- Aspartame
- Sucralose
- acesulfame K

- saccharin
- xylitol
- sorbitol
- erythritol
- high-fructose corn syrup
- glucose
- fructose
- Golden syrup
- Agave syrup
- Rice malt syrup

Fats & Oils

All industrial seed oils such as:

- vegetable oil
- canola oil
- cottonseed oil
- rapeseed oil
- corn oil
- sunflower oil
- hydrogenated oil
- safflower oil
- soybean oil
- peanut oil
- Non-extra virgin olive oils
- margarine and spreads
- Lard
- Shortening

Drinks

• All soda drinks, energy drinks, and diet

sodas

• Commercial fruit juices and smoothies

(even raw)

• Fruit cordials

• Milkshakes and flavored milk

• Artificial alcoholic beverages

• Soya milk

Fruits

• All fruit that is high in sugar

Grains

All grains, gluten, and flours:

- Wheat
- corn,
- rice
- spelt
- rye
- buckwheat
- barley
- oats
- bulgur

Other foods to avoid:

- beans

- lentils

- Peanuts

- Grain-fed meat and dairy

- All grains

- Soy

- Potatoes

My experience with alkaline-keto diets

To be honest, at first, I felt guilty about eating all those fats...and using full-fat products.

I thought to myself, won't it make me fat?

It took me a while to break through my old beliefs, and what was helpful was continuous education about the keto diet. That kept me very motivated.

I was already familiar with a clean food diet based on alkaline, paleo, and Mediterranean diets. But the keto element was definitely new to me, and I had to learn how to use fats and which fats to eliminate.

For example:

<u>Fats to avoid:</u>

-industrial seed oil, trans fatty acid

- industrial vegetable oil they are very processed, very corrosive to our arteries, they produce heart disease

-Soybean oil

-Sunflower oil

-Cottonseed oil

-Corn oil

-Canola oil (rapeseed oil)

Condiments like mayonnaise also contain the above-mentioned toxic oils and so do industrially made bakes and goods.

The fast food industry uses those oils too.

The common mistakes with the ketogenic diet:

The most common mistake that people make is that they do not include enough veggies with their keto foods. That can cause imbalance and acidity. Hence, I am such a big fan of keto and alkaline diets combined together. Green vegetables are a fantastic addition to your keto diet.

They will help you have more energy and also add more variety to your diet.

The real keto lifestyle is about variety, abundance, and energy. It's hard to be successful with a keto diet if a menu consists entirely of animal products.

The role of alkaline foods

It's important to get a ton of greens and alkaline foods as these foods are rich in minerals and vitamins while at the same time don't contain sugar.

I have been promoting alkaline foods for years.

They oxygenate your body and help you have more energy and can be combined with other diets such as paleo or keto diet.

In its optimal design, alkaline diet advocates using good plant-based oils such as avocado and olive oil, and coconut oil and it also excludes wheat products and crappy carbs.

Foods that are rich in sugar are also excluded. The alkaline diet includes low sugar fruits (limes, lemons, grapefruits etc.)

One of the main principles of the alkaline diet is adding a ton of green veggies into your diet.

The best way to be adding these alkaline foods is via veggie smoothies and juices. The recipe section of this book will give you some ideas. There are also many fantastic alkaline friendly drinks that will not only help you re-energize and alkalize your body without messing around with your keto lifestyle but will also bring more variety into your diet. Many of these drinks will help you feel more relaxed and balanced.

They will also help you quit drinking sugary drinks, and soda's and in many cases can also help you reduce your caffeine intake. It's a great feeling if you can just wake up and go without depending on caffeine and sugar and feeling moody all the time.

How long to feel the benefits? For most people, it takes a few days to a couple of weeks. It all depends on where you are right now. However, do not get too distracted to compare yourself to other people.

What about exercise? Is it essential on an alkaline keto diet?

The answer is both yes and no. It depends on what you mean by the word "exercise."

For example, many people think they can get away with eating a poor, processed diet, by working out beyond their limits and throwing some supplements on top of that.

And, it works. Many people neglect what they eat, and still enjoy good looking bodies, because of their working out routine. The problem? It's not very sustainable. And most people can get away with in their early twenties.

Unfortunately, eventually, abusing their bodies with constant acidity, sugars, crappy carbs, and even some aggressive supplements will catch on.

One of the sad lessons I learned (I used to be obsessed with fitness and over-exercising), is that fitness does not always equal to health.

What you really want to focus on is a balance. Real fitness comes from how healthy you are and how you feel.

In other words- you can't outwork a bad diet...

However, physical activity is essential. Luckily, it doesn't have to be complicated. Just move your body every day. It can be a short walk. It can also be a short home workout. You can look for simple, 10-

minute body-weight workouts and do them before work. They will help you burn fat during your working hours and give you a fantastic sense of accomplishment).

Since our goal is a profound transformation and a lifestyle change, I highly recommend you pick just one physical activity you really enjoy and commit to it. Even 5 minutes a day is better than nothing. Getting started with such a mindset will help you create a habit.

You can slowly build up on your working out routine from there.

Whenever I am really pressed for time, I just set my timer for 5 minutes, play my one of my favorite songs and do some squats and push-ups. I also use this technique when I feel lazy, and guess what, moving my body helps me get rid of that laziness, and usually, I end up wanting to work out more and more.

The basic rule is always- don't overthink it, just do something to move your body.

You can also start by walking. Daily walks are really amazing for your overall health. Personally, I love walking combined with listening to audiobooks. I get a fantastic sense of accomplishment- I am learning, relaxing, and getting some exercise and oxygen at the same time.

And it's fun, you don't need any equipment, and it's cheaper than going to the gym. However, the gym could be a good idea if you are working from home, or simply need a break, or perhaps you really need the gym environment to get pumped, that's fine too.

The basic rule is: Start experimenting to figure out what works for you.

A healthy diet is much more important than going to the gym on a poor diet, and so, that should be your priority.

Luckily, by transitioning your diet to a more alkaline-keto friendly diet, you will have more energy and that energy will make you want to move your body.

Before we dive into the recipes, we would like to offer you a free access to our VIP Wellness Newsletter

www.yourwellnessbooks.com/email-newsletter

Here's what you will be receiving:
-healthy, clean food recipes and tips delivered to your email
-motivation and inspiration to help you stay on track
-discounts and giveaways
-notifications about our new books
-healthy eating resources to help you on your journey

No Fluff, no spam. Only good and easy to follow info!

Sign up link (copy this link to your phone, or PC):

www.yourwellnessbooks.com/email-newsletter

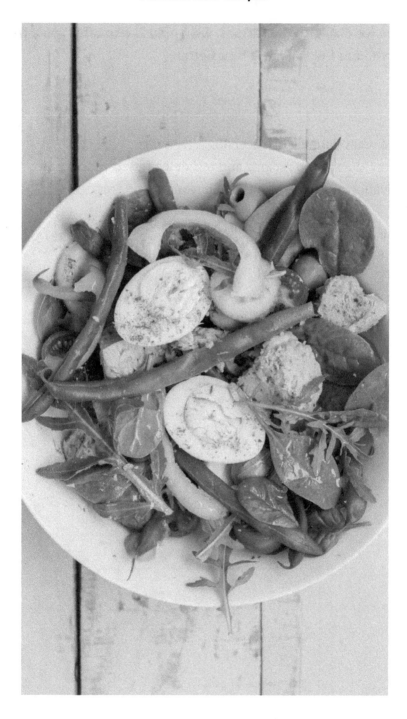

About the Recipes-Measurements Used in the Recipes

The cup measurement I use is the American Cup measurement.

I also use it for dry ingredients. If you are new to it, let me help you:

If you don't have American Cup measures, just use a metric or imperial liquid measuring jug and fill your jug with your ingredient to the corresponding level. Here's how to go about it:

1 American Cup= 250ml= 8 Fl.oz.

For example:

If a recipe calls for 1 cup of almonds, simply place your almonds into your measuring jug until it reaches the 250 ml/8oz marks.

I hope you found it helpful. I know that different countries use different measurements, and I wanted to make things simple for you. I have also noticed that very often those who are used to American Cup measurements complain about metric measurements and vice versa. However, if you apply what I have just explained, you will find it easy to use both.

Alkaline Keto Recipes

When it comes to alkaline keto recipes, there is no need to organize or categorize them into breakfasts, lunch, or dinner. The reason is simple- many recipes can be served both for dinner and breakfast. And some dinner leftovers can also be turned into a quick take away lunch.

Following this "philosophy," I decided to organize the recipes into:

-healthy smoothies and soups:

These are great for all kinds of occasions and are just perfect if you don't have the time to cook. A nutritious vegetable smoothie with good fats in it will help you stay full for hours, and it is terrific meal replacement. At the same time, many smoothies can be transformed into a delicious, healing soup. With herbs, spices, and Himalaya salt, they will taste amazing. You can also add in some boiled eggs, fish, or some meat leftovers. It's effortless to create a healthy "meal" while on this lifestyle.

Alkaline keto soups can also be served as a side dish, and they always get people's attention.

-easy salads:

These can be both raw and cooked and are a great option as take away meals. If you are pressed for time, it's so easy to quickly put some alkaline keto friendly foods together and make a "little" salad that will help you stay full for hours. I used to worry that eating a salad will not keep me full, but I was wrong. I also feared I would miss carbs and snacks in between my meals. Once again, I was wrong. Alkaline keto salads are so balanced they will keep you full and nourished for hours. Good, healthy fats and a myriad of greens and other healthy superfoods will eliminate all unhealthy food cravings. The truth is that you crave what's in your blood. So, if you keep adding sugar and crappy carbs, your body will want more and more of it. Luckily, by focusing on healthy, alkaline keto foods, you will finally fell free from unwanted sugar cravings, and so, you will feel empowered to eat in a healthy, balanced, nourishing way.

-satisfying meals:

Ok, so this recipe section includes the recipes that my mom calls "normal food"). Eggs and bacon, delicious fish, warm, satisfying recipes for breakfast, lunch, and dinner, and much, much more...yummy!

-alkaline keto drinks:

These are great to sip on in between your meals to take care of your hydration as well as vitamin and mineral intake. I will show you my favorite tea and herbal tea recipes, including my alkaline keto bulletproof hormone rebalancing tea. You will love it! I will also show you other alkaline keto approved tonics to take care of your hydration. You will no longer feel tempted to drink sugary drinks and sodas...You already know they can get you out of balance.

Luckily, these recipes will help you make the transition.

-fresh alkaline keto approved juices:

These are absolutely phenomenal if your goal is to lose weight and stay energized. The primary purpose of alkaline keto juices is to add in more alkaline foods to your diet. It may be hard to eat all those greens and veggies, and so, many people find it easier to juice them and then just sip on their green juices in between their meals. This is a very healing, juicing therapy, and it will also help you have healthy looking skin, shiny hair, and strong nails. You will be getting a ton of easy to absorb nutrients and vitamins with no sugar and no carbs. Also, pure, fresh green juices can be added to your soups or bone broths. Whenever I make chicken soup, I like to add in 1 cup of raw kale or spinach juice. I am always on a mission to add more greens to my diet, and it just works so well.

-alkaline keto snacks:

If you can't live without snacks, don't worry, you are in for a guilt-free treat! The best stuff comes at the end of this booklet...

Alkaline Keto Nourishing Soups and Smoothies

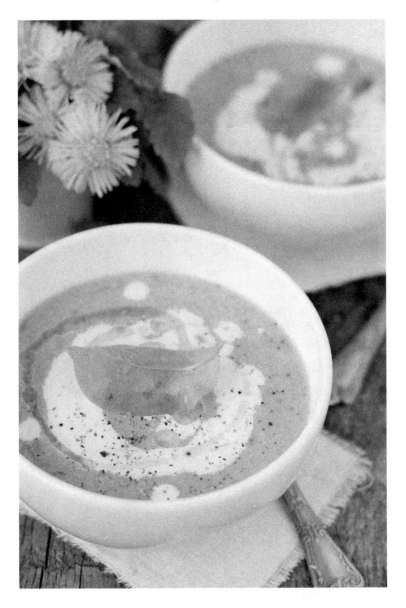

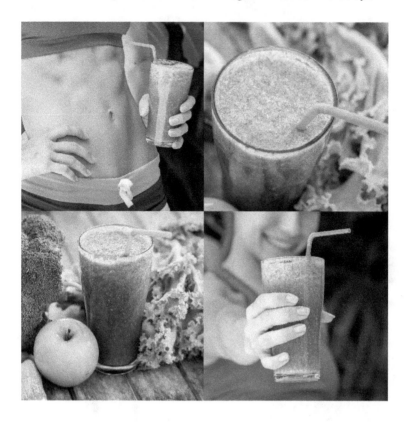

Green Dream Weight Loss Smoothie

This green vegetable smoothie blends the best of the alkaline and keto worlds. It's my number one recommendation if your goal is weight loss and energy. It may take some time to get used to green vegetable smoothies, especially if you are used to drinking sweet fruit smoothies (not good for you, unfortunately).

But trust me, after a few green smoothies, and a fantastic energy they provide, you will be wondering how you could ever live without them.

Himalaya salt really makes it taste delicious. Now, I like to keep my recipes as simple as possible, without too many ingredients.

But to let you know the variations of this recipe- you could also add in some cilantro, curry and chili pepper if you like spicy smoothies.

If you go for this variation, you may also heat up the smoothie and serve it as a beautiful, warm soup (and add some coconut or other full fat creams on top). Enjoy!

Servings: 2

Ingredients:

- 1 cup coconut or almond milk (unsweetened)
- 1 cup water (filtered, preferably alkaline)
- 1 small avocado, peeled and pitted
- A handful of spinach
- 1 tablespoon coconut oil or flaxseed oil
- Pinch of Himalaya salt to taste

Instructions:

1. Place all the ingredients in a blender.
2. Blend well.
3. Serve and enjoy!

Easy Spicy Veggie Smoothie

This smoothie will help you enrich your diet with healthy, alkalizing vegetables. I like to make this smoothie in the evening and use one serving as a quick detox soup (yea, you can heat it up a bit) and then I keep the second serving as a quick morning smoothie.

Servings: 2

Ingredients:

- 1 green bell pepper
- 1 small avocado, peeled and pitted
- 1 small garlic clove, peeled
- Pinch of black pepper and chili
- 1 cup water (filtered, or alkaline water)
- 1 tablespoon extra-virgin olive oil
- Himalaya salt to taste

Instructions:

1. Place all the ingredients in a blender.
2. Process until smooth, serve, and enjoy!

Coconut Almond Balancer

This delicious smoothie uses stevia (both alkaline and keto friendly natural sweetener) so that you can enjoy an excellent, creamy sweet taste.

It also uses maca powder, which is a hormone re-balancer for women.

Enjoy!

Ingredients:

- 1 cup coconut milk, unsweetened
- A handful of almonds (raw, unsweetened and soaked in filtered, alkaline water for a few hours)
- 1 tablespoon coconut oil
- A bit of stevia to sweeten
- Half teaspoon fresh maca powder

+ a few lime slices and ice cubes to serve if needed

Instructions:

1. Place all the ingredients in a blender.
2. Process until smooth.
3. Serve and enjoy!
4. This smoothie also tastes delicious when chilled or half frozen.

Vitamin C Alkaline Keto Power

This delicious smoothie is jam-packed with vitamin C coming from alkaline and keto friendly fruits like limes and lemons.

Now, I understand that looking at the ingredients of this recipe, you may be feeling a bit "turned off." Yes, alkaline keto smoothies are very different to usual "sweet fruity smoothies".

But, give it a try. It tastes great! Very similar to natural, Greek yogurt.

You can also use this smoothie recipe to season your salads. Most salad seasonings are full of crappy carbs, sugars and a ton of chemicals, while this smoothie is 100% natural!

Another suggestion is - you could use this smoothie recipe to make a smoothie bowl by adding in some protein of your choice.

Once you have tried this smoothie, you will get my point for sure!

Servings: 2

Ingredients:

- 1 big avocado, peeled, pitted and sliced
- Half lemon, peeled and sliced
- 1 cup of coconut milk
- 1 teaspoon coconut oil
- Pinch of Himalaya salt
- Pinch of black pepper
- A few slices of lime to garnish

Instructions:

1. Place all the ingredients in a blender.
2. Process until smooth.
3. Serve in a smoothie glass and garnish with a few lime slices.
4. Drink to your health and enjoy!

Hormone Rebalancer Natural Energy Smoothie

This smoothie recipe is a fantastic option if you don't like green smoothies, but you still want to experience all the health benefits of alkaline keto smoothies.

This recipe uses stevia which is a natural sweetener, very often used both on keto and alkaline diets.

Although, let me remind you that once your taste buds have adapted, you will be able to do without any sweeteners easily.

Still, if you need one- go for stevia.

Servings: 1-2

Ingredients:

- 1 big grapefruit, peeled and halved
- 1 cup water (filtered, preferably alkaline)
- 1 inch of ginger, peeled
- 1 tablespoon coconut oil
- Half teaspoon maca powder
- Stevia to sweeten, if desired

Instructions:

1. Blend all the ingredients in a blender.
2. Serve and enjoy!

Green Mineral Comfort Smoothie Soup

This recipe can be used both as a smoothie as well as a soup.

Whenever I am pressed for time, I make it for dinner, to enjoy something warm and keep the raw leftovers to have a nourishing green smoothie in the morning.

Servings: 1-2

Ingredients:

- 1 big cucumber, peeled
- 1 small avocado, peeled and pitted
- A handful of parsley
- A handful of cilantro
- 1 cup of thick coconut milk
- A handful of raw cashews
- 1 tablespoon of olive oil
- Himalaya salt to taste
- 1 chili flake

Instructions:

1. Blend all the ingredients in a blender.
2. Serve raw as a smoothie, or heat it up (using low heat) and serve as a gentle, detox, comforting soup.
3. Enjoy!

White Creamy Buttery Soup

This super easy recipe needs only 5 ingredients (seasonings included).

It's perfect if you crave something creamy. My secret addiction (for many years) was bread with butter. And, for years I was convinced it was the bread I wanted. However, after transitioning my diet to a more keto friendly lifestyle, I realized I no longer crave bread. All I need is a little butter!

This recipe also uses healing alkaline veggies like cauliflower, and, at the same time, adds in some garlic to help you strengthen your immune system.

Servings: 1-2

Ingredients:

- 1 cup cauliflower, slightly cooked or steamed, cut into smaller pieces
- 4 tablespoons organic butter (you can also use coconut oil instead)
- 1 cup water (filtered, preferably alkaline)
- 2 garlic cloves, peeled and minced
- Himalaya salt

Instructions:

1. In a small pot, combine the butter and garlic.
2. Fry the garlic on low heat.
3. Cover.
4. In the meantime, using a blender, combine the cooked cauliflower, 2 pinches of Himalaya salt and water.
5. Now add the mixture to the pot with butter and garlic.
6. Simmer on low heat until the soup is warm and creamy.
7. If needed, add more Himalaya salt to taste (as well as other spices if desired).
8. Serve and enjoy.

Suggestion- if you want to add in some protein, you can use some fried bacon or hard-boiled eggs.

You could also add in some goat cheese (it's a great treat as well!), and /or chia seeds.

Anti-Flu Mediterranean Keto Smoothie Soup

This is another, super easy recipe that you can enjoy both as a quick, raw smoothie, or a beautiful, healing soup (raw or slightly cooked).

It's full of anti-inflammatory properties, and it also helps fight colds and flu.

Servings: 1-2

Ingredients:

- 4 medium-sized tomatoes, peeled
- 1 big garlic clove, peeled
- 4 small celery sticks
- 2 tablespoons olive oil
- A handful of black olives
- Half cup water, preferably alkaline (or filtered water)
- Himalaya salt to taste
- 1 teaspoon oregano
- A few fresh basil leaves
- 1 hard-boiled egg (optional)

Instructions:

1. Combine all the ingredients in a blender.
2. Process well until smooth. Add more water if needed.
3. Serve in a smoothie or soup bowl and add in a hard-boiled egg.
4. Serve and enjoy!

Alkaline Keto Super Easy Salads

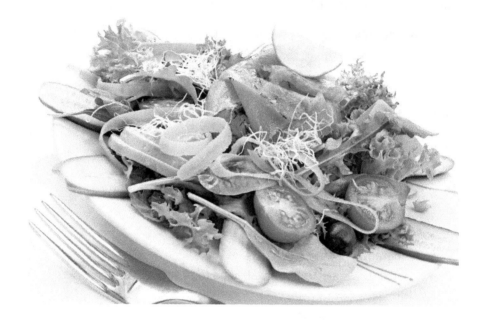

Almost Sushi Alkaline Keto Salad

I used to be addicted to sushi. And there is nothing wrong with that, as long as you go out for sushi as a treat. But in my case, I was really getting hooked on it.

As a result, I was putting on weight. Unfortunately, most sushi restaurants use a myriad of seasonings that are high in carbs, sugar, and calories.

And so I asked myself- is there something easy I could make at home that could offer me a similar "sushi experience"?

Luckily there is. I realized that what I really craved was the taste of nori.

And, it's very easy to use it in a salad, alongside with fresh avocado and smoked salmon as well as some alkaline greens.

Nori is an excellent source of Iron as well as Omega 3 Fatty Acids and vitamins A & C., And it tastes so delicious in salads!

Servings: 1-2

Ingredients:

- 4 slices of fresh, smoked salmon
- 1 big avocado, peeled, pitted and sliced
- 2 big nori sheets, cut into smaller pieces
- 2 cucumbers, peeled and sliced
- 2 tablespoons avocado oil
- 2 tablespoons fresh lime or lemon juice
- Himalaya salt to taste

Instructions:

1. Combine all the ingredients in a small salad bowl.
2. Add the Himalaya salt, avocado oil, and some fresh lime (or lemon juice).
3. Serve and enjoy!

Green Power Plants Salad

This salad can be prepared in 2 different versions- vegetarian or with meat.

Servings: 2-3

Ingredients:

Salad Base:

- 1 cup arugula leaves, washed
- 1 small avocado, peeled, pitted and sliced
- 2 cucumbers, peeled and sliced
- 1 tablespoon fresh lemon juice
- 2 tablespoons olive oil
- Himalaya salt and black pepper to taste

Option 1- Vegetarian

2 hard-boiled eggs (shell removed)

A few (fat) slices of goat cheese

Option 2 – Meat or Fish

Half cup of any meat or fish leftovers you have (chicken, beef, salmon).

Instructions:

1. In a big salad bowl, combine all the ingredients from the "salad base."
2. Sprinkle with lemon juice and olive oil.
3. Add Himalaya salt. Toss well.
4. Now add in the rest of the ingredients of your choice (option 1 or 2, or both if you like).
5. Serve and enjoy!

Irresistible Vegetarian Mediterranean Salad

This salad is perfect if you are pressed for time and are looking for a quick and healthy way to put a nice, nourishing meal together.

Servings: 2

Ingredients:

- 1 cup of mixed greens
- 2 tomatoes, sliced
- A few onion rings
- 6 big slices of goat cheese (preferably organic)
- A few slices of avocado
- Half cup of green olives
- 1 can of tuna (organic)
- 1 tablespoon lemon juice
- 2 tablespoons olive oil (organic)

Instructions:

1. Mix all the ingredients in a big salad bowl.
2. Sprinkle with olive oil and lemon juice.
3. Toss well, serve and enjoy!

Easy Creamy Warm Salmon Salad

Salmon is definitely one of my favorite keto ingredients, especially to use for quick, nourishing salads like this one.

Servings: 1-2

Ingredients:

- Half cup raw cashews, crushed
- 4 slices of smoked salmon
- 2 tablespoons of coconut oil or butter
- 1 cup fresh spinach
- 2 tomatoes, sliced
- Himalaya salt and black pepper to taste
- A few thin slices of cheddar cheese

Instructions:

1. Place coconut oil in a frying pan.
2. Switch on the heat (medium heat).
3. Add the spinach and Himalaya salt and stir-fry until soft.
4. Now, add the salmon, cashews and tomato slices.
5. Stir fry until the salmon is warm.
6. Take off the heat and place in a salad bowl.
7. If needed, add more Himalaya salt to taste.
8. Top up with some cheddar cheese, serve and enjoy!

Alkaline Keto Protein Salad

Eggs can be a real lifesaver, especially for quick alkaline keto salads that are rich in protein.

I like to boil the eggs in bulk, to make sure I always have 1 or 2 to add to my salad.

Servings: 1-2

Ingredients:

- 2 hard-boiled eggs, peeled
- 1 cup of mixed greens of your choice
- A few onion springs
- 1 green bell pepper, sliced
- 1 small avocado, peeled and pitted
- 1 small garlic clove
- 2 tablespoons olive oil
- 2 tablespoons water

Instructions:

1. Combine the eggs and greens in a salad bowl.
2. Add the onion springs.
3. Now, using a small hand blender, blend the avocado, with olive oil, water and Himalaya salt.
4. Spread the avocado dressing onto the salad, toss well, serve and enjoy!

Arugula Vitamin C and A Salad

This simple salad is very rich in Vitamins C and A, as well as healthy Omega's and of course- good fat-burning fats!

Grapefruit is a fantastic fruit that is both alkaline and keto friendly. It's because, it is full of alkaline minerals like magnesium and potassium, while at the same time it's a low sugar fruit. Exactly what we want on this diet and lifestyle!

Servings: 1-2

Ingredients:

- Half cup fresh parsley
- 1 grapefruit, peeled
- 1 cup arugula leaves
- Half avocado
- 1 can of organic tuna
- Himalaya salt to taste
- 2 tablespoons of avocado or olive oil

Instructions:

1. Combine all the ingredients in a salad bowl.
2. Toss well, serve and enjoy!

Bacon Easy Keto Salad

This salad is just perfect for all the bacon lovers out there.

The "secret sauce" here are greens and veggies that help create balance!

Servings: 1-2

Ingredients:

- A few slices of bacon, fried in butter or coconut oil
- 2 tomatoes, sliced
- Half avocado, peeled and sliced
- 1 cup of kale leaves, washed and chopped
- 1 small garlic clove, peeled and minced
- A few greens and black olives (optional)
- Himalaya salt to taste
- Half lemon

Instructions:

1. Combine all the ingredients in a salad bowl.
2. Sprinkle with some fresh lemon juice and Himalaya salt.
3. Serve and enjoy!

Easy Balancing Delight Salad

This salad uses fennel, which is a very alkalizing ingredient (it's naturally sweet and delicious). It combines really well with coconut milk, cashews, and avocado, offering a simple, entirely plant-based alkaline keto salad that is great for detox, or as a side dish.

Ginger is an amazing addition to this salad- it's full of anti-inflammatory properties and also helps strengthen the immune system.

Enjoy!

Servings: 1-2

Ingredients:

- 1 fennel bulb cut into smaller pieces
- A handful of cashews
- Half avocado, peeled and sliced
- Half cup thick coconut milk
- 1 tablespoon avocado oil
- Pinch of Himalaya salt
- 1 teaspoon grated ginger
- 2 tablespoons chive

Instructions:

1. Place all the ingredients in a salad bowl.
2. Sprinkle with oil, coconut milk, and salt.
3. Toss well, serve and enjoy!

Low Carb Spaghetti Spicy Salad

This salad is full of good fats, alkalizing veggies, delicious taste, and optimal hydration.

Perfect as a quick dinner!

Servings: 2

Ingredients:

- 2 medium-sized zucchinis, spiralized (if you don't have a spiralizer, just cut them into super thin slices)
- A handful of fresh cilantro leaves
- 3 slices of smoked salmon, cut into smaller pieces
- Half teaspoon black pepper
- Half teaspoon Himalaya salt
- Half teaspoon curry powder
- Half teaspoon ginger powder
- 3 tablespoons coconut oil

(optional): serve with 1 cup fresh arugula leaves and 1 avocado and lime

Instructions:

1. Put a frying pan or a pot on low heat.
2. Add the coconut oil, spices, and salt.
3. Add the spiralized zucchini and stir well.
4. Keep stir-frying until soft.
5. Now, add the smoked salmon and cilantro and stir-fry on a low heat for a few minutes.
6. Turn off the heat and cover for a few minutes.

7. In the meantime, in a small salad bowl, prepare a side salad by combining the arugula leaves with avocado slices, Himalaya salt, and lime.

Now, transfer the spiralized zucchini with salmon to a big plate (or 2 plates), serve and enjoy together with arugula salad.

Chicken Curry Salad

This recipe is just perfect if you have some chicken leftovers in your fridge and fancy a quick, warm, refreshing salad.

Servings: 1-2

Ingredients:

- 1 cup shredded chicken
- 1 cup spinach leaves
- 2 tablespoons coconut oil
- A pinch of chili powder
- Half teaspoon curry powder
- Himalaya salt to taste
- 2 big tomatoes, sliced

Instructions:

1. In a frying pan, combine the coconut oil and spinach.
2. Put on low heat, and keep stirring while adding the spices and salt.
3. Once the spinach gets soft, add the chicken.
4. Keep stir-frying on allow heat for several minutes.
5. Allow the chicken to absorb the oil and spices.
6. Switch off the heat.
7. Serve with the raw, sliced tomatoes.
8. Enjoy!

Keto Friendly Super Delicious Satisfying Meals (with plenty of alkaline foods)

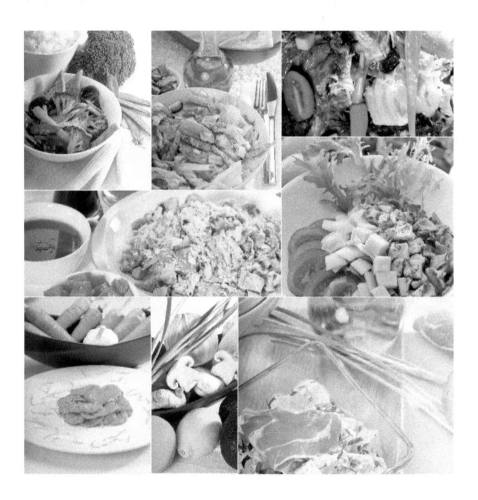

Easy Low Carb Pizza Adventure

Yes, you heard me right. You can enjoy a healthy homemade pizza on this lifestyle. And...you can use it to add in some alkaline veggies too!

This recipe is just perfect for a lovely, lazy weekend evening when you're feeling cozy watching movies (keep the leftovers for the next day, pizza for breakfast, every now and then is also a great idea!).

Please note- this recipe calls for a processed ingredient (tortillas). For me, personally, it's OK occasionally. However, if you're looking for a 100% keto friendly recipe that will provide very similar taste experiences, I recommend you try the following recipe in this book (Irresistible Veggie Pizza) and skip this one.

Servings: 2
Ingredients:

- 2 tablespoons coconut oil or organic butter
- 2 tablespoons olive oil
- 2 large low-carb, gluten-free tortillas
- 6 tablespoons organic tomato sauce (you can also make your own by blending 1 tomato with 1 tablespoon olive oil)
- 1 green bell pepper, minced
- 2 cans of natural tuna
- 1 cup shredded mozzarella cheese
- 4 teaspoons dried Italian seasoning
- Pinch of Himalaya salt

Instructions:

1. Using a large skillet (over medium-high heat) heat the coconut oil.
2. Add the tortilla.
3. Using a spoon, spread the tomato sauce over the tortilla.
4. Then, add the cheese, the seasonings, salt, tuna, and veggies.

5. Cook until crispy and then place on a cutting board and cut into thin slices.
6. Sprinkle with 1 tablespoon of organic olive oil on top.
7. Repeat the process to make more if needed.

Suggestions:

The possibilities are endless with this recipe. Feel free to experiment by adding veggies, greens, smoked salmon, some meat leftovers...whatever you want.

You can use all kinds of organic cheeses, veggies, and if desired, some meat or fish.

Irresistible Veggie Pizza

This is a delicious vegetable-based dish that combines the benefits of alkaline keto diets. It also calls for good fats while helping you enjoy the aroma and taste of cheese and Italian spices.

Servings: 4

Ingredients:

- 4 big zucchinis, peeled and cut lengthwise, very thin
- 4 tablespoons coconut oil
- 2 red bell peppers
- 2 green bell peppers
- 1 big onion, peeled and cut into thin rings
- 1 cup mushrooms, washed and sliced
- 1 cup mozzarella cheese powder
- Half cup organic tomato sauce (or blend 2 tomatoes with 2 tablespoons of olive oil to make your own)
- Himalayan salt
- 1 tablespoon oregano

Instructions:

1. Pre-heat the oven to 500 °Fahrenheit (or 260 °Celsius).
2. Grease a big, flat baking dish with coconut oil.
3. Add the zucchini and then the successive layers of red and green bell peppers, mushrooms and onions.
4. Sprinkle the cheese, salt, and oregano.
5. Place in the oven for about half an hour.
6. Serve and enjoy!

Simple Spicy Egg Scramble

This recipe is perfect as a tasty, energizing breakfast or a quick meal.

Feel free to experiment with all kinds of spices for this one. Personally, I love chili powder!

Servings: 1-2

Ingredients:

- 2 tablespoons coconut oil
- Half cup shredded chicken
- 6 eggs
- 2 tablespoons coconut cream or thick coconut milk
- Pinch of chili powder
- Pinch of Pink Himalayan salt
- Pinch of freshly ground black pepper
- ½ cup shredded cheese
- Half cup green bell pepper, sliced
- A handful of chopped chive and dill

Instructions:

1. In a large skillet over medium-high heat, melt the coconut oil.
2. Add the chicken and sauté for 5 minutes until cooked.
3. In a separate bowl, whisk the eggs until frothy.
4. Now add the cream, salt, and spices.
5. Whisk to blend thoroughly.
6. Add the egg mixture to skillet with chicken and heat (on low heat) until almost cooked through, about 4 minutes.
7. When the eggs are almost done, add in shredded cheese and bell pepper.
8. Serve hot with some fresh chives and dill.

Turkey Broccoli Mix

This recipe proves how delicious and healing the alkaline keto mix can be.

Good fats, lean protein, and green veggies really help your body thrive and transform on a deeper level.

Servings: 2-3

- 6 turkey slices (thin)
- 1 small broccoli, cut into small florets, steamed or lightly cooked
- 4 garlic cloves, minced
- 1 small onion, diced
- 4 large eggs
- 2 tablespoon olive oil,
- Pink Himalayan salt
- Freshly ground black pepper

Instructions:

1. In a large skillet over medium-high heat, stir-fry the turkey slices in coconut oil (for about 2)

2. Turn the heat down to medium, and add the steamed broccoli florets, garlic, and onion.

3. Sautee for a few minutes.

4. When the veggies get tender, add the eggs by scrambling them all over the skillet. Keep stir frying until the eggs are set.

5. Sprinkle the olive oil on top, and serve hot.

Kale Avocado Vegetarian Combo

This recipe combines the best of the low carb, vegetarian, alkaline and keto diets. And it's so easy to make! Even if you are pressed for time.

Servings: 1-2

Ingredients:

- 2 tablespoons coconut oil
- 2 cups zucchini slices
- Half cup kale, chopped
- 1 avocado, sliced
- 4 large eggs
- Pinch of Pink Himalayan salt
- Pinch of Freshly ground black pepper
- Optional: a pinch of red chili powder

Instructions:

1. In a large skillet, heat 1 tablespoon of coconut oil.
2. Add the zucchini, and sauté on medium heat for about 3 minutes.
3. Add the salt and spices.
4. In the meantime, "massage" the kale with the remaining 1 tablespoon of coconut oil so that it gets tender.
5. Add the kale to the skillet on top of the zucchini slices.
6. Now, add the avocado slices on top of the kale.
7. Using a spoon, create a space for the eggs.
8. Add the eggs.
9. Cover the skillet and cook for about 5 minutes (or until the eggs are done)
10. Serve hot and season with more spices and Himalaya salt if needed.
11. Enjoy!

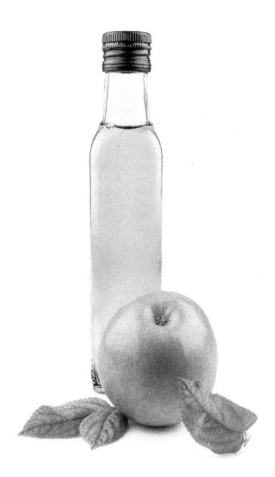

Alkaline Keto Drinks (to help you have more energy!)

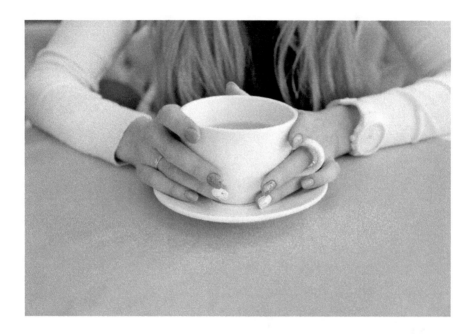

Ginger and Turmeric Hormone Balancing Bulletproof Tea

This tea is excellent for getting rid of coughs and colds and will perform wonders for those looking to lose excess weight. It blends good fats with nutrition and alkalizing herbs.

Since there is no caffeine in this tea, you can enjoy it whenever you want, even in the evening.

Serves: 1

Ingredients:

- 2-inch ginger, peeled
- 2-inch turmeric, peeled
- 1 cup water, boiling
- 1 tablespoon coconut oil
- A pinch of Ashwagandha powder
- 2 slices of lime

Instructions:

1. Place all the tea ingredients (except coconut oil and Ashwagandha) in a teapot and pour over some boiling water.
2. Keep covered for 15 minutes.

3. Strain and serve warm (but not boiling) in a teacup with coconut oil and lime slices. Stir in the Ashwagandha powder and stir again, enjoy!

Easy Chili Tea

This tea will help in cleansing your digestive tract while warming you up and giving you a substantial energy boost that will last for hours.

Serves: 2

Ingredients:

- 2 cups water, boiling.
- 2 Rooibos tea bags
- 2 red chili flakes
- A handful of fresh mint leaves
- 2 tablespoons coconut oil or organic butter

Instructions:

1. Place all the tea ingredients (except coconut oil) in a teapot and pour over 2 cups of boiling water.
2. Keep covered for 15 minutes.
3. Strain and serve warm (but not boiling) in a teacup with coconut oil or butter.

Cumin and Caraway Tea

This tea is excellent for those women looking to obtain relief from period cramps. Adding in some good fats enhances the therapeutic properties of this alkaline keto style tea.

Serves: 1-2

Ingredients:

- 2 cups water, boiling
- 1-inch ginger, peeled
- 1 tablespoon cumin seeds
- 1 tablespoon caraway seeds
- 1 tablespoon coriander seeds
- 1 tablespoon fennel seeds
- 2 tablespoons coconut oil or avocado oil

Instructions:

1. Place all the tea ingredients (except the oil) in a teapot and pour over 2 cups of boiling water.
2. Keep covered for 15 minutes.
3. Strain and serve warm (but not boiling) in a teacup with the coconut or avocado oil.

Spicy Chai Tea

This tea is super tasty and creamy. It's great to prevent colds too. It's one of my favorite comfort, alkaline keto teas!

Serves: 1-2

Ingredients:

- 1 cup almond or coconut milk
- 1 Indian chai tea bag
- 2-inch turmeric, peeled
- 1-2 chili flakes
- 1 tablespoon coconut or olive oil

Instructions:

1. Boil almond milk using a saucepan.
2. When boiling, add the tea bag and turmeric.
3. Simmer on low heat for 5 minutes.
4. Turn off the heat and keep covered for 15 minutes.
5. Pour into a teacup and add in the oil.

***In the absence of chai tea, make use of tea leaves mixed with cinnamon, cloves, and cardamom.

Ashwagandha Alkaline Keto Tea

This is an excellent tea for those looking to increase their immunity and balance. Personally, I like this tea at nighttime as it helps me sleep like a baby.

Serves: 1-2

Ingredients:

- Half teaspoon dried Ashwagandha
- 2 cups water, boiling
- 1 chamomile tea bag
- 1 fennel tea bag
- 1 tablespoon coconut oil

Instructions:

1. Place all the tea ingredients (except the coconut oil) in a teapot and pour over some boiling water.
2. Keep covered for 15 minutes.
3. Strain and serve warm (but not boiling) in a teacup with 1 tablespoon of coconut oil.

Sleep Well Alkaline Keto Tea

This recipe will help you unwind after a busy day, sleep like a baby, and wake up feeling energized. The cinnamon powder makes this tea naturally sweet, without compromising it's no sugar alkaline keto friendly guidelines.

Serves: 2

Ingredients:

- 1 cup of water, boiling
- 1 lemongrass stalk
- 2 tablespoons chamomile tea
- A few tablespoons of coconut milk
- 1 tablespoon of coconut oil
- A dash of cinnamon powder to garnish

Instructions:

1. Place all the tea ingredients (except coconut milk and oil) in a teapot and pour over some boiling water.
2. Keep covered for 15 minutes.
3. Strain.
4. Pour into a teacup and add in the coconut milk and oil.
5. Stir well.
6. Sprinkle over some cinnamon powder, enjoy!

Easy Mediterranean Anti-Inflammatory Tea

This tea can be made in 2 different ways:

1. You can choose to add in some green tea, if you need more energy, for example, if you are using this tea in the morning.

2. You can choose to add in some Melissa tea, if you need to unwind, for example, if you are using this tea in the evening and want to relax and sleep well.

Rosemary and fennel are both miraculous herbs and will help you boost your immune system and fight off colds and flu.

Fennel is also great for weight loss as well as stimulating your lymphatic system.

Serves:2

Ingredients:

- 2 cups boiling water
- 1 tablespoon rosemary herb
- 1 tablespoon fennel seeds
- 1 teaspoon green tea, or Melissa tea (optional)
- 1 tablespoon olive oil

Instructions:

1. Place all the tea ingredients (except the oil) in a teapot and pour over some boiling water.
2. Keep covered for 15 minutes.
3. Strain and serve warm (but not boiling) in a teacup with 1 tablespoon of olive oil.

Lime Refresher Alkaline Iced Tea

Blueberries are known for their antioxidant providing abilities, and they are wonderfully sweet. Add the addition of spicy herb and a lime twist, and you have a hydrating drink that is alkaline-keto friendly.

Ingredients

- 2 grapefruits, peeled and sliced
- 2 limes, peeled and sliced
- 1 medium bunch of fresh oregano
- 1 liter of water – filtered if liked

Instructions

1. Pour the water into a suitable container or jug.
2. Add the grapefruit slices to the water, squashing a third of them on to a plate beforehand, and catching any juice to add too.
3. Juice one of the limes and add the juice to the water. Slice the other lime into thin pieces.
4. Wash the oregano and give it a bit of a "squeeze" to start releasing some of its flavor.
5. Add the herbs to the water and mix really well. Leave in the fridge for at least an hour before serving.

Fresh Alkaline Keto Approved Juices (to help you get back in balance)

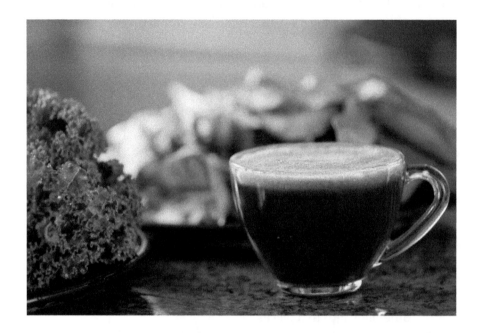

Health benefits of using Alkaline Keto Juices include:

- You give your digestive system a rest
- You get more energy
- It's easier to juice a mountain of fresh greens and veggies than to eat them
- Great for weight loss- you give your body a myriad of vitamins and nutrients with literally no calories. Your body gets hydrated and energized , and so you no longer crave unhealthy foods or sugars.

Juicing vs. Smoothies? What is the Difference?

You are probably wondering what is better for you. Juicing vs. Smoothies? The answer is – both are amazing.

It all depends on your health goals and personal preferences.
Juicing is an excellent option for people who want to increase their intake of fresh veggies and greens, but their digestive systems are too sensitive to handle massive amounts of fiber.

So, in this case, juicing is excellent! With juicing, you can get benefits of awesome produce without suffering any stomach issues for your juicing efforts.

Juices are natural to digest and easy to assimilate form.

The golden rule is- when juicing, focus on:

-all kinds of veggies and greens that can be juiced

-low sugar fruit (for example lemons, limes, pomegranates, grapefruits)

Tips for getting started with juicing:

- Prepare your House: Clean out the fridge and pantry and be sure it's stocked with tons of fresh and frozen produce.

- Begin by adding a handful or so of organic baby spinach into your juices, especially if you're new to green juices.

- Invest in a good juicer and set an intention (for example: "I can't wait to get started on this journey and to juice 3 times a week" – is a simple to follow through goal and intention).

- Prepare all your juices the night before and store them in air-tight containers for the following day. Making all the juices at once can save time in clean up and ensures you're ready with fresh juice whenever needed.

- There are so many variations of Juicing, you can use the recipes and add or take away ingredients. Feel free to swap for your favorite ingredients, just make sure you're getting a tasty variety throughout the day.

The juicer I like to use is Omega Juicer. However, any other cold pressed juicer will do.

Make sure you wash all the ingredients before you proceed to your juicing rituals.

Now, back to the recipes!

Cucumber Kale Alkaline Keto Juice

While it's hard to eat a mountain of greens and cucumbers, it's easy to drink their juice and get all the vital nutrients in. Avocado oil offers good fat to help you absorb the minerals and vitamins from the juice.

Servings: 2

Ingredients:

- 1 lemon, peeled
- 3 celery stalks, chopped
- A couple dashes of hot habanero sauce
- a handful of kale, chopped
- 2 big cucumbers, peeled and chopped
- a drizzle of avocado oil
- Himalaya salt to taste
- Optional: 1 cup of water (filtered or alkaline)

Instructions:

1. Place through a juicer.
2. Juice.
3. Pour into a glass and add in a couple dashes of hot habanero sauce, if needed.
4. You can also dilute this juice in water.

5. Enjoy, you are drinking health and energy!

Easy Flavored Spinach Juice

While pure spinach juice can be a bit hardcore, this recipe is a bit different.

Add in some fresh ginger and mix it with coconut milk and oil, and you will fall in love with green juice.

One green juice a day will keep the doctor away!

Serves: 2

Ingredients:

- 2 cups of fresh spinach
- 2-inch ginger, peeled
- 1 tablespoon melted coconut oil
- 1 cup of coconut milk

Instructions:

1. Place the spinach and ginger through a juicer.
2. Extract the juice, pour it in a big glass.
3. Combine with coconut milk and oil.
4. Stir well and enjoy.

Red Bell Pepper Antioxidant Juice

Red bell pepper, ginger, and healing greens is an excellent combination.

It makes the juice taste nice and helps you get accustomed to juicing greens.

Servings: 2

Ingredients:

- 1 big red bell pepper, chopped
- 1 cup mixed greens of your choice (I like to throw in some spinach, arugula, and mint)
- 2 inch of ginger, peeled
- 2 tablespoons avocado or olive oil
- Himalaya salt to taste

Instructions:

1. Juice all the ingredients using a juicer.
2. Serve in a glass.
3. Enjoy!

Simple Lemon Tonic

This "juicy tonic" helps maintain a healthy digestive system.
Mix it with some water if needed.

Servings: 2

Ingredients:

- 2 cups of mint leaves, chopped
- 2 grapefruits, peeled and chopped
- 1 lemon, peeled and halved
- 1 inch of ginger, peeled
- 1-inch turmeric, peeled
- 2 cups of water

Instructions:

1. Place all the ingredients in a juicer.
2. Juice.
3. Combine with 2 cups of water, using a water jar.
4. Serve chilled with some ice cubes.
5. Enjoy!

Alkaline Keto Hydration Mineral Green Juice

This is a super hydrating juice that is full of energy restoring alkaline minerals and healthy fats. Perfect for a hot day when you need to take care of your energy levels, quickly, effectively, and naturally.

Servings: 2

Ingredients:

- 4 big cucumbers, peeled and chopped
- 2 zucchinis, peeled and chopped
- 2 limes, peeled and chopped
- 1 big romaine lettuce
- 1 tablespoon olive oil
- Himalaya salt to taste

Instructions:

1. Place all the ingredients through a juicer.
2. Extract the juice.
3. Pour into a chilled glass and enjoy!

Easy Tasty Green Juice

Red bell peppers are one of my favorite veggies to juice.

They are naturally sweet and full of vitamins and minerals. They

make any green juice taste amazing. Ginger adds to anti-

inflammatory properties.

Servings: 2-3

Ingredients:

- 1 cup celery, chopped
- 3 red bell peppers, chopped
- 1 inch of ginger, peeled
- 2 slices of lime, to garnish
- 2 tablespoons coconut oil
- 1 cup of coconut milk
- 1 teaspoon cinnamon powder
- Fresh ice cubes

Instructions:

1. Juice all the ingredients using a juicer.
2. Pour in a glass, add in some ice cubes.
3. Mix with coconut milk and coconut oil.
4. Garnish with lime slices.
5. Serve and enjoy!

Totally Guilt Free Alkaline Keto Snacks

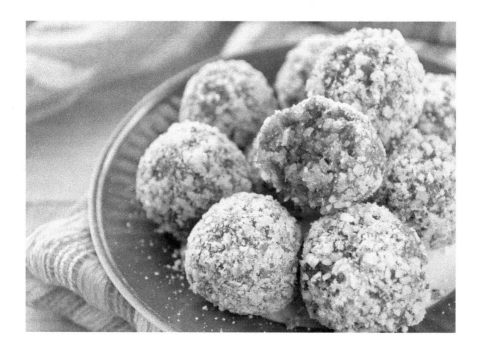

Ridiculously Easy Sweet Alkaline Keto Balls

This recipe is a must-try to help you:

-satisfy your "sweet tooth" without eating crappy carbs or sugars

-add in some good fats and anti-inflammatory properties too

-sneak in some alkaline keto superfoods to make sure you stay energized

Ingredients:

- 1 cup raw cashews (unsalted, unsweetened), soaked for at least 4 hours
- 1 cup raw almonds (unsalted, unsweetened), soaked for at least 4 hours
- 4 tablespoons coconut oil
- 4 tablespoons coconut milk
- 1 tablespoon cinnamon powder

Instructions:

1. Place all the ingredients in a high-speed blender or a food processor.
2. Using your hands, form the "dough" into small balls.
3. Place the balls on a big plate and put in a fridge for a few hours.
4. Serve and enjoy!

Creamy Sweet Alkaline Keto Porridge

This recipe is perfect if you are craving something sweet and creamy. It's super easy to make.

Servings: 2

Ingredients:

- 1 cup raw cashews
- 1 cup of coconut milk
- 2 tablespoons coconut oil
- 1 tablespoon cinnamon powder
- 1 tablespoon chia seeds
- Optional: 1 teaspoon maca powder
- A few blueberries to garnish

Instructions:

1. Combine all the ingredients in a bowl.
2. Mix well, serve and enjoy!

Delicious Chia Pudding Recipe

I came up with this recipe by accident. Just using the ingredients, I had available. To my surprise, the result was really delicious (and super healthy). This guilt-free treat is loaded with fiber, Iron, calcium, and omega-3 fatty acids. After all, chia seeds are one of the most nutritious foods on the planet and are just perfect for treats, smoothies and all kinds of creamy recipes.

Servings: 2

Ingredients:

- 1 cup unsweetened full-fat coconut milk
- Half teaspoon liquid stevia to sweeten (it's optional though, you can do very well without it)
- Half teaspoon vanilla extract
- Half teaspoon cinnamon powder
- Half cup fresh blackberries, preferably organic
- 4 tablespoons chia seeds
- Optional: half teaspoon maca powder
- Optional: half teaspoon ginger powder

Instructions:

1. Process all the ingredients using a blender or a food processor.
2. If needed, process a few times, to make sure you obtain a smooth mixture.
3. Now, divide the mixture between two small cups with lids, and refrigerate overnight (or, for at least a few hours).
4. Serve and enjoy, it's really delicious!

Pure Mint Choco Guilt-Free Ice Cream

Nothing compares to fresh, homemade, low carb, nutrient-packed ice-cream! Oh, and to make this recipe, you don't need any fancy ice cream maker. Not at all!

Servings: 2

Ingredients:

- 2 tablespoons coconut oil or butter
- 1 teaspoon stevia
- 10 tablespoons heavy (whipping) cream,
- Half teaspoon peppermint extract
- 4 tablespoons sugar-free dark chocolate chips

Instructions:

1. In a small, heavy saucepan melt the butter or coconut oil (using medium heat)
2. Now, add in the stevia and 5 tablespoons of cream.
3. Bring the mixture to a boil, and keep stirring.
4. Now, turn the heat down to low and simmer, for about 30 minutes.
5. Simmer occasionally and turn off the heat once the mixture gets thick.
6. Add in the peppermint extract and stir well.
7. Pour the mixture into a bowl and place in a fridge to cool.
8. In the meantime, pour the remaining 5 tablespoons of cream into another bowl.
9. Whip the cream, so it gets thick and fluffy.
10. Take the cream mixture out of the refrigerator and place the whipped cream into the cooled mixture.
11. Add the chocolate chips.

12. Now, put the mix in a small container, cover, and place in a freezer (make sure the container you are using is suitable for this "mission").
13. Freeze for about 6 hours before serving.
14. Serve and enjoy!

Amazing Keto Chocolate Shake

Who said that a healthy lifestyle means no desserts?

You can enjoy desserts in a homemade, healthy, clean version. You have already learned how to make super healthy salads and smoothies, and it's all great. But we only live once, and so whenever you crave a shake, enjoy this one! No sugars, no nasty chemicals...

Servings: 2

Ingredients

- 1 cup heavy (whipping) cream, or coconut cream
- Half cup coconut milk (or almond milk) unsweetened
- 1 teaspoon stevia
- Half teaspoon maca powder
- Half teaspoon vanilla extract
- 4 tablespoons unsweetened cocoa powder

Instructions:

1. Pour the cream into a chilled metal bowl.
2. Start beating the cream with a hand mixer.
3. Keep beating until it forms peaks.
4. Stir in the coconut milk.
5. Proceed to add stevia, maca, cocoa, and vanilla powder.
6. Beat again until the mixture is thoroughly combined.
7. Pour into shake classes and chill in a fridge for a couple of hours.
8. Serve and enjoy!

Suggestions: you can serve the shake with some protein powder or chia seeds.

Eating Out While on Alkaline Keto Mix Lifestyle

Good news, my Dears!

It's actually very easy.

1. If possible, check the restaurant's menu online, before booking.

(although this is not always necessary as even most "normal" restaurants will have alkaline keto foods on their list).

2. Go for a big, green salad (perfect as an appetizer) with some fish or meat. Or just a vegetable salad with olive oil. You could also indulge in a little bit of cheese. Another option is – meat or fish with vegetables (no potatoes).

3. Be sure to avoid any processed salad dressings. Instead, ask for a raw salad with some olive oil, spices, and lemon juice.

4. As for drinks, order water with lemon, or herbal infusion. Most restaurants do offer herbal teas.

5. Occasional treats like a glass of wine, expresso, or even a little dessert are absolutely fine. Although I would keep treats only for special social occasions.

6. Most restaurants will be pleased to customize their menu and services to your needs, so don't be shy, always ask if they can re-modify some of their meals for you. It's as simple as getting rid of that sugar and carb filled salad salsa or getting rid of potatoes and artificial seasoning to make your meal more alkaline-keto friendly.

Questions:

You can email me at:

info@yourwellnessbooks.com

We Need Your Help

One more thing, before you go, could you please do us a quick favor?

It would be great if you could leave us a short review on Amazon.

Don't worry, it doesn't have to be long. One sentence is enough.

Let others know your favorite recipes and who you think this book can help.

Your opinion is important.

Thank You for your support!

Join Our VIP Readers' Newsletter to Boost Your Wellbeing

Would you like to be notified about our new health and wellness books?

How about receiving them at deeply discounted prices? And before anyone else?

What about awesome giveaways, latest health tips, and motivation?

If that is something you are interested in, please visit the link below to join our newsletter:

www.yourwellnessbooks.com/email-newsletter

It's 100% free + spam free, and you can easily unsubscribe whenever you want.

We promise we will only email you with valuable and relevant information, delicious recipes, motivational tips, and more!

Sign up link:

www.yourwellnessbooks.com/email-newsletter

More Books by Elena Garcia:

www.amazon.com/author/elenagarcia

More Books & Resources in the Healthy Lifestyle Series

These books are available on Amazon in eBook, paperback and audiobook format

You will find them by looking for *Elena Garcia* in your local Amazon store, or by Visiting:

www.yourwellnessbooks.com

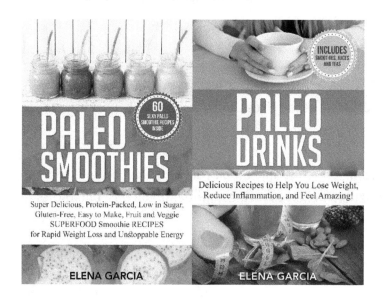

CPSIA information can be obtained
at www.ICGtesting.com
Printed in the USA
LVHW082102080920
665324LV00016B/478